- Studi[...] magn[...] [...]in (B₁) deficiencies—try spinach, avocados, and almonds for magnesium, asparagus and whole wheat bread for thiamin.

- Put a few drops of lavender oil on your pillow.

- Avoid antihistamines several hours before bedtime.

- Keep the lights off during those middle-of-the-night bathroom trips.

You'll find practical tips like these—plus scientific facts about sleep and a list of helpful resources—in . . .

101 WAYS TO FALL ASLEEP

101
Ways to Fall Asleep

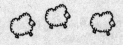

Nancy Butcher

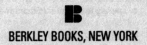

BERKLEY BOOKS, NEW YORK

101 WAYS TO FALL ASLEEP

A Berkley Book / published by arrangement with the author

NOTE: Every effort has been made to ensure that the information contained in this book is complete and accurate. However, neither the publisher nor the author is engaged in rendering professional advice or services to the individual reader. The ideas, procedures, and suggestions contained in this book are not intended as a substitute for consulting with your physician. All matters regarding your health require medical supervision. Neither the author nor the publisher shall be liable or responsible for any loss, injury, or damage allegedly arising from any information or suggestion in this book. The opinions expressed in this book represent the personal views of the author and not of the publisher.

PRINTING HISTORY
Berkley edition / August 2002

Copyright © 2002 by The Berkley Publishing Group
Book design by Julie Rogers
Cover design by Rita Frangie

Visit our website at
www. penguinputnam.com

ISBN: 0-425-18576-1

BERKLEY®
Berkley Books are published by The Berkley Publishing Group, a division of Penguin Putnam Inc., 375 Hudson Street, New York, New York 10014.
BERKLEY and the "B" design are trademarks belonging to Penguin Putnam Inc.

PRINTED IN THE UNITED STATES OF AMERICA

10 9 8 7 6 5 4 3 2

CONTENTS

INTRODUCTION

Why Aren't We Getting More Sleep?

*I am so anxiety-ridden all the time that I stay up
really late worrying about stuff, so that by the time
I force myself to go to bed, I'm so exhausted that I
fall asleep immediately. But I have to wake up
early, so I'm constantly tired, in any event.*

—Amanda, age 33*

*I almost never sleep more than four to six hours
per night. As a result, I am what my wife calls
"pathologically exhausted," and I never have problems falling asleep. That's true even when I wish I
did—I've fallen asleep walking the dog, eating,
commuting by bus to work (waking up back where
I started rather than where I was going), and talking on the phone. When I drink coffee at night, it
doesn't keep me up; it helps me wake up the next
morning.*

—Ron, age 42

---

*Many people contributed anecdotes to this book. In order to protect
their anonymity, their real names were not used.

Sleep—it's a wonderful thing. What could be better than snuggling under the covers at the end of a long, hard day, closing your eyes, and enjoying eight hours of uninterrupted rest, rejuvenation, and happy dreams?

Unfortunately, for Amanda and Ron and millions of others, good sleep is an elusive holy grail. According to the National Sleep Foundation's 2001 Sleep in America poll[†]:

- 63 percent of American adults do not get the recommended eight hours of sleep per night.

- 31 percent reported sleeping less than seven hours on weeknights, although some of them tried to catch up on the weekends—a practice that can actually perpetuate the bad-sleep cycle.

- 22 percent of adults claim that they are so sleepy during the day that it interferes with their activities for a few days, a week, or longer.

These statistics show that almost a quarter of us— and some experts suggest that this number is much higher—are going to work, raising children, and in

----

[†]To check out the rest of the 2001 Sleep in America poll, go to the National Sleep Foundation's Web site at *www.sleepfoundation.org*.

general leading our lives in a state of perpetual exhaustion.

What is wrong with this picture?

Why aren't we getting more sleep?

INSOMNIA NATION

Insomnia is a major culprit. According to experts, an estimated 40 million people suffer from this sleep disorder, which can be defined as:

- Having trouble falling asleep at night

- Waking up in the middle of the night and tossing and turning

- Waking up too early in the morning and not being able to get back to sleep

- Waking up feeling tired and unrefreshed

Insomnia can be a condition in and of itself that may be related to lifestyle, diet, sleep habits, age, and more. It can also be a side effect of certain prescription or over-the-counter medications such as painkillers, sedatives, and antihistamines, or a symptom of a physical or psychological ailment.

Besides insomnia, there are other sleep disorders that affect the quality and duration of sleep—and lead to other health problems as well. Examples include obstructive sleep apnea, a potentially life-threatening condition in which the sleeper stops breathing for brief periods of time, and restless leg syndrome (RLS), in which the sleeper experiences aches, pains, tingling, itching, or other uncomfortable sensations in the legs, accompanied by an almost irresistible urge to move them. And of course, there is good old-fashioned snoring, which can wake *everyone* up.

TOO BUSY TO SLEEP

Another enemy of sleep is our crazy-busy, 24/7 culture. As many of us try to juggle full-time-plus careers, families, social lives, civic lives, and more, sleep becomes less a priority and more a thing to be "squeezed in" between other, more pressing activities.

According to the Sleep in America poll, 40 percent of adults report that they spend more time at their jobs than they did five years ago; 38 percent say they work fifty hours or more per week. Coincidentally, 38 percent say they spend less time sleeping. The poll concludes that those who work more sleep less—and also experience more insomnia.

In theory, sleep should be as fundamental to us as food, water, and air, and getting *good* sleep should be at the top of our to-do lists. But in practice, it is often at the bottom.

THE COSTS OF TOO LITTLE SLEEP

We are paying for our ongoing sleep debt—in spades. Poor sleep can have a host of negative consequences on our health, safety, and well-being. It can lead to illness. It can cause car accidents. It can impair our memory and productivity. It can make us irritable and moody. It can take a terrible toll on our relationships.

If that isn't bad enough . . . evidence suggests that sleep deprivation might actually make us grow older faster. In a study published by the October 1999 issue of *Lancet,* researchers at the University of Chicago reported disrupting the sleep of eleven young men—all healthy—over the course of six nights. The researchers concluded that sleep deficit can have a negative impact on carbohydrate metabolism and endocrine functions, similar to the changes that take place during the aging process.

Unlike Rip Van Winkle, who grew old while he slept, many of us may be experiencing accelerated aging while we're *not* sleeping.

WHAT HAPPENS DURING SLEEP, ANYWAY?

Contrary to popular belief, we are very *busy* during sleep. While we're "just lying there," there are all kinds of fluctuations happening in our brain waves, body temperature, respiration, heart rate, muscles, and more. And all this nocturnal activity plays a major role in energizing and rejuvenating our bodies; helping our brains acquire, process, store, and retrieve information; and regulating immune, cardiovascular, and other functions.

Sleep consists of several stages, characterized by changing brain-wave activity and other factors:

▪ *Stage 1 Sleep:* This is the "theta wave" stage of sleep, in which you begin to relax and your breathing begins to slow. During this "half-asleep" time, some people wake up momentarily with a jerk. It can last up to ten minutes.

▪ *Stage 2 Sleep:* This stage, which might last ten to twenty minutes, is considered by most sleep experts to be the beginning of "real sleep."

▪ *Stage 3 Sleep:* During this stage, which can last about the same amount of time as Stage 2, your muscles are very limp, and your breathing is even. If you are awakened during this stage, you may feel disoriented.

▪ *Stage 4 Sleep:* During this stage—often called "delta sleep," because of the delta-wave activity in your brain—you are in your deepest sleep state, not unlike hibernation. It is very difficult to wake people up during Stage 4 sleep. It can last for half an hour or so.

▪ *REM ("Rapid Eye Movement") Sleep:* This very active stage is characterized by rapid eye movements as well as increased pulse, respiration, blood pressure, body temperature, blood flow to the brain, sexual arousal, and other physical changes. During this stage, you are likely to experience your first dream of the night.

During a continuous night of sleep, you will go from Stage 1 to 2, 3, and 4—then back up through 3 and 2. But instead of reverting all the way back to Stage 1, you will go through a REM stage—after which you will go back to a cycle of 2, 3, 4, 3, and 2. And then you will start at REM and go through the 2, 3, 4, 3, 2 cycle all over again. So one night of sleep would look roughly like this:

YOU GO TO BED
    Stage 1
    Stage 2
    Stage 3
    Stage 4
    Stage 3
    Stage 2
      REM Stage
    Stage 2
    Stage 3
    Stage 4
    Stage 3
    Stage 2
      REM Stage
AND SO ON UNTIL YOU WAKE UP IN THE MORNING

As the night goes on, the length of your REM stage tends to increase. And because the REM stage is considered to be highly beneficial in terms of your daytime physical and mental functioning, the longer you sleep, the longer and more frequent your REM stages will be.

HOW MUCH SLEEP DO WE REALLY NEED?

Most experts agree that the average adult needs eight hours of sleep per night. Some experts even argue that we need ten for optimal daytime functioning and performance.

On the other hand, there are some who suggest that we need as much sleep as we *believe* we need, and that the barometer should be how we feel and function during the day. In other words, if you're doing just fine with six hours per night, then perhaps that is all you need.

A lot of it has to do with your heredity. If your parents didn't require much sleep to function optimally, you may not, either.

In any case, take a long, hard look at your sleep habits—and at your life. Do you need an alarm clock to wake up? Do you hit the snooze button several times because you just want to "sleep for a few more minutes"? Do you feel groggy and drowsy during the day? Are you less than productive at work? Are you chronically cranky and irritable?

Then you need more sleep!

WHEN TO SEE YOUR DOCTOR

If your sleep problems are prolonged and/or are seriously interfering with your daily activities; if you think you suffer from a sleep disorder such as sleep apnea or restless leg syndrome (RLS); or if you suspect that your sleeplessness stems from an underlying medical condition or a medication side effect, first make an appointment to see your doctor. He or she will be able to provide an accurate diagnosis and prescribe the appropriate treatment. Medical conditions and symptoms that can lead to sleep problems include (but are not limited to):

- Depression

- Anxiety disorders

- Heart disease

- Respiratory problems

- Cancer

- Arthitis and other conditions characterized by joint or muscle pain

- Nighttime heartburn

- Hypertension

- Menopause/night sweats

- Chronic fatigue syndrome

- Seasonal affective disorder (S.A.D.)

- Overactive thyroid gland

- Allergies

- Impotence

- Urinary, gastrointestinal, or other conditions that necessitate trips to the bathroom in the middle of the night

In general, if you are having problems sleeping, you may want to see your doctor first to rule out any of the above. Your doctor can also recommend a sleep specialist or a sleep clinic if he or she feels that it would be beneficial.

HOW TO USE THIS BOOK

Once your doctor has given you a clean bill of health—or if you don't need to see the doctor at all but simply want to *start sleeping better*—then read on. You're about to discover 101 ways to do just that.

The first chapter in this book—"The Perfect Bedroom"—will help you set up just the right environment for you to get your zzz's.

Subsequent chapters will take you chronologically through your day and night so you can get the best sleep possible. First, there's "Good Daytime Habits for Good Nighttime Sleep." Then there's "As the Sun Goes Down...," which offers tips on what to eat for dinner and when, how to create a regular winding-down routine, and more. "Time for Bed!" will tell you just what to do when you're ready to turn in. The chapter "If You're Up in the Middle of the Night" will help you get back to sleep if you're up at 2 A.M. tossing and turning.

Finally, there are special chapters with tips on trying to sleep with a newborn or small children in the house; trying to sleep with a noisy or restless partner; pregnancy-related sleep problems; coping with jet lag; coping with shift work; whether or not to take sleeping pills; and more.

As you go through this book, try to identify the things that may be causing your sleepless nights. Are you chronically stressed out? Do you smoke? Do you drink too much caffeine? Does your job involve frequent shift changes? Do you have a lumpy mattress? Do you carry the weight of the world on your shoulders? Do you live in a noisy neighborhood? Do you like your alcohol? Are you overweight? Do you watch violent TV shows late at night? Do you and your partner argue in bed? There are many factors that can contribute to insomnia that may surprise you.

Hopefully, by the time you've made it through all 101 tips, you will be well on your way to a new way of sleeping—a way that will enhance your health, well-being, productivity, mood, and more.

And now, happy reading—and sweet dreams!

The Perfect Bedroom

Remember the story of "The Princess and the Pea"? A bedraggled-looking young woman shows up at a prince's castle, claiming to be a princess. She asks for a bed for the night—a pretty major bed, consisting of twenty mattresses, each one stacked on top of the other.

In order to test the woman's claim of royal heritage, the prince places a pea under the very bottom mattress. The next morning, when he asks her how she slept, she complains: "I couldn't sleep. There was a lump in my bed!" The prince concludes that such a sensitive creature must surely be of royal blood!

The moral—at least for the purposes of *this* book, anyway—is that in order to get a good night's sleep, it's essential to have a good bed, a good bedroom, and more. Here are eighteen tips to achieve just that.

1. Make your bedroom a haven.

Think of your bedroom as the place for the three R's: retreat, relaxation, and rest. (No, make that

I used to use my bed as my desk. I did work there, E-mail, everything, and soon I began to dread going to bed. Instead, I'd hit the couch and end up waking up all cranky. Then I made a rule: No work-related stuff in the bedroom. It's made all the difference.

—Amy, age 25

four: romance!) Your bedroom should be your sanctuary from the world. That means no piles of bills on the nightstand . . . no ironing board in the corner overflowing with wrinkly clothes . . . no fax machine beeping and spitting out documents all night. If you live in a small apartment or house and your bedroom must serve double or triple duty, hide all evidence of Real Life in closets, storage boxes, or pretty containers at the end of each day.

2. Pick peaceful colors.
Choose soothing colors for your walls and bedding, like cream, pale yellow, peach, pink, lavender, light green, or sky blue. Or simply pick your favorite colors—but stay away from jarring ones like magenta or lime.

3. Be a kid again.

Some people find it comforting to re-create details from their childhood bedrooms. How about the wallpaper pattern you grew up with? A mobile? A big, fuzzy teddy bear? Glow-in-the-dark stars for your ceiling?

A string of tiny lights wrapped around your bedpost? A Lava lamp? Hey, even your autographed Donny Osmond poster? If that helps.

4. Buy the right mattress.

A quality mattress is one of the best investments you can make for good sleep, good health, and more. You can choose from standard coil mattresses or foam mattresses. Foam mattresses, which include "futon"-style mattresses, tend to be less expensive but not as long-lasting. With either coil mattresses or foam mattresses, the issue of firmness is crucial. Thin people (i.e., those of us with little natural padding) or elderly people with painful conditions such osteoporosis and arthritis might prefer a softer mattress. Almost everyone else—especially those of us with lower-back problems—will want a firmer mattress.

5. When you go shopping for a mattress, make sure to take it for a "test drive."

Here's how:

▪ Kick off your shoes and lie flat on your back. Does the mattresss feel deliciously comfortable and cozy, like you could take a nap right there in the store?

▪ Roll onto your side with your arms at your sides. You should experience no discomfort in your arms, shoulders, or hips while you do this.

▪ Bounce up and down on every single inch of the mattress. It should feel consistently resilient but supportive.

▪ If two of you will be sharing the mattress, test-drive it together. (But keep it G-rated!)

6. Remember that size matters!
Does your sleeping situation make you think of "Goldilocks and the Three Bears"? ("This bed is too big!" "This bed is too small!") When you select a mattress, make sure there's enough room for you and any sleeping companions, including significant others, children, and pets. It's better to err on the side of too much room—you can always snuggle in the middle.

7. Choose the rest of your bed wisely.
If you're buying a coil mattress, consider buying the box spring at the same time—they often come in

---

According to the Better Sleep Council:

A **twin-sized** mattress is approximately
38 × 74.5 inches.

A **full-sized** mattress is approximately
53 × 74.5 inches.

A **queen-sized** mattress is approximately
60 × 79.5 inches.

A **king-sized** mattress is approximately
76 × 79.5 inches.

"sets" and are designed to work together. You will also need a frame and possibly a headboard, depending on your needs. A foam mattress will require some sort of platform bed. Some people prefer sleeping close to the floor, on only a mattress.

8. Dress your bed well.

If you've always wondered what the heck "percale" is, you're about to find out. Percale is a tightly woven cotton cloth used commonly for bedsheets. The cotton is often blended with polyester, and sometimes with silk or linen. The higher the thread count, the finer and more durable the fabric. As an alternative to percale,

---

Water beds, which were popularized in the 1960s, are still around today. Many of them have a groovy system that keeps the sloshing and wave action to a minimum. If you're considering buying a water bed, remember that it will require a lot of floor support. It will also have to be heated in the winter.

---

cotton flannel sheets are wonderful, especially in the cold months. Linen sheets, while expensive, will help keep you cool in the summer. My personal year-round favorites are "jersey" sheets—the cotton is really soft, like a favorite old T-shirt. Silk and satin sheets are sexy, but they may feel too cold and slippery for sleeping purposes. You be the judge.

9. Find a pillow that fits.

When it comes to pillows, you have a vast menu to choose from. First, there is the natural-versus-synthetic option. Natural pillows are filled with goose down and feathers, and are lovely, warm, and comfy. They are also expensive, and can trigger allergic reactions in some people. The more down, the softer; the more feathers, the firmer. Synthetic pillows are less pricey and also have the advantage of washability; however, they tend to be on the thin side. There are also various "contour pillows" for people with back, neck, and special sleep issues.

10. Cover up—but not too much.

It's important to have just the right number of blankets (and quilts and comforters) when you sleep. Otherwise, you will find yourself waking up in the middle of the night because you're too hot or too cold, or because you're playing blanket tug-of-war with your partner. One option to consider is an electric blanket, which comes with individual controls on each side. You can also get electric blankets with specialized "heat zones"—warmest at the foot of the bed, less warm in the middle, and least warm at the top. A final note: If you're allergic to wool, steer clear of blankets with wool fiber content.

11. Indulge in a security blanket.

Remember how nice it was to have a security blanket as a child? Consider buying an *adult* security blanket (or quilt or afghan) that you can wrap around yourself at night. Like the one in your childhood, it will not only comfort you but provide a practical association: Blankie means bedtime.

12. Take care of your bed.

Some (but not all) new mattresses should be turned and rotated periodically to prevent wear and tear—ask your salesperson or manufacturer. Evaluate your mattress once a year or so and make sure it's still providing you with the support and comfort you need. Like anything else, mattresses do wear out. Vacuum your mattress to keep it free of dust, pet hair, and the like.

13. Take care of your bedding.

Launder sheets and pillowcases at least weekly, and all other bedding—quilts, blankets, comforters, dust ruffles, etc.—at least monthly. And remember to make your bed every day. It's much nicer to have a tidy, pretty bed to retreat to every night (rather than a messy, chaotic jumble of blankets and sheets).

14. Set your thermostat.

The ideal temperature for sleeping is sixty to sixty-five degrees Fahrenheit. For the summer months, you should have an air conditioner or a fan.

15. Don't dry out.

The humidity in your bedroom should be around 60 to 80 percent. A too-dry bedroom will dry out your skin, nose, and throat, making it hard to sleep. A humidifier in your bedroom can help. Conversely, if your bedroom is *too* humid, you will feel—well, too sweaty and yucky to sleep. If this is the case, you will want to get yourself a dehumidifier or an air conditioner.

16. Ventilate!
If weather permits, keep your windows open while you sleep so you can get fresh air. If not, consider buying an overhead fan that will keep the air moving (and also create a romantic Southern ambience).

I am addicted to my white-noise machine . . . so much so that if the power goes out and it turns off, I wake up! It seems not only to soothe me but block out aberrant noise.

—Sylvia, age 44

---

17. Say no to noise.
Noise—whether from loud neighbors, sirens, or garbage trucks—is the enemy of sleep. To make your bedroom a temple of restful silence, think

White noise machines create a constant, fuzzy, soothing noise that covers up undesirable noises by producing a mix of soundwaves over a wide frequency. Some machines also offer other comforting sounds, such as the sound of rain, waterfalls, or shushing waves. Machines are available at stores like the Sharper Image and Brookstone; check ads or go on-line. Prices can range from around fifty to two hundred dollars. Some people prefer buying white-noise or soothing-noise CDs and programming them to play all night.

about investing in thick carpeting (which absorbs sound) and double-pane windows. Heavy drapes can also help cut down on the din from outside. Air conditioners and fans can provide a lulling "white noise" effect to drown out other unwanted noises. Or better yet, you can purchase a white-noise machine.

18. Get rid of annoying or distracting appliances.

In the spirit of keeping the bedroom the bedroom, remove the TV. Also remove any office machines.

If you have a ticking clock, switch to an electric, nonticking one. If you have an electric clock with a bright or blinking LED, switch to one with a less glaring display.

Good Daytime Habits
for Good Nighttime Sleep

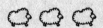

Your falling-asleep routine shouldn't start after the sun goes down. It should start the second you wake up. Indeed, what you do during the daylight hours will very much affect how you sleep—or don't sleep—at night.

It's all about what you put into your body, how you manage stress, how you tackle your to-do list, and more. An added plus: If you incorporate these good-for-you habits into your daily routine, you'll improve not only your sleep patterns but your overall health, wellness, and well-being. What more can you ask for?

19. Wake up at the same time every morning!

Starting tomorrow, decide on a good wake-up time that will work for you—6 A.M., 7 A.M., 8 A.M.— and stick to it. Do this every morning, no exceptions—even if you are up until 3 A.M. watching *Star Trek* reruns. In a few weeks, your body will adjust accordingly, and you will find yourself getting drowsy at about the same time every night.

It's okay to wake up earlier once in a while—e.g., to catch a flight or make a breakfast meeting. Just don't wake up later.

20. Don't sleep in on weekends.
Many people do this because they think they're "making up" for bad sleep during the week. But in truth, this practice will throw off your internal clock and disrupt your sleep patterns even more. It can also lead to the phenomenon known as "Sunday-night insomnia."

21. Start waking up earlier gradually.
If you decide that you want to start waking up at 7 A.M.—but you're used to getting up at 8 A.M.—then set your clock a few minutes earlier each day until you're getting up ten to fifteen minutes earlier every morning.

22. If possible, wake up without an alarm clock.
This will enable you to wake up when your body's natural clock dictates. If you're concerned about accidentally oversleeping, use the alarm clock as a backup.

23. Have a wake-up routine every morning.
Establish a routine that will help you greet the day with joy and optimism. Some suggestions:

Good Daytime Habits for Good Nighttime Sleep

▪ Cue your clock radio to play your favorite station or CD—Alanis Morissette, the soundtrack from *Fame,* whatever gets you going.

▪ Open the window and let the sun in.

▪ Count your blessings.

▪ Do some long, luxurious stretches in bed.

▪ Meditate for ten minutes, breathing deeply from the center of your belly and letting any and all thoughts flow out of your head.

▪ Take a hot shower with soaps and shampoos containing peppermint, eucalyptus, and other energizing scents.

▪ While you get dressed, look up your horoscope on the Internet.

▪ Write one E-mail message—just one—to someone you love.

▪ Then write another one to yourself with a cheerful (or goofy) message for the day, and send it to your office E-mail address so it will be waiting for you.

I start each day with a prayer. It gives me a positive boost and sets the tone for the rest of the day.

—Beth, age 40

24. Eat a healthy diet.

The average American diet is not a sleep-friendly diet. If you're used to eating a lot of meat, refined carbohydrates, and rich, high-fat foods, start replacing them *right now* with whole grains, legumes, veggies, and fruits. And instead of eating a small breakfast (or worse, no breakfast at all), a big lunch, and a gigantic dinner, reverse the order—and throw in some nutritious, satisfying snacks. Start with a hearty breakfast of oatmeal or other whole-grain cereal, nonfat yogurt, skim milk, and gads of fresh, seasonal fruit. Have a whole-wheat muffin with marmalade or a boiled egg for a midmorning snack. For lunch, make a yummy sandwich on whole-wheat bread with your favorite combination of fillings—choose from skinless broiled chicken, low-fat cheese, veggies, nonfat mayo, honey mustard, relish. Soup is also terrific—as long as you stay away from the cream-based kind. Satisfy the midafternoon munchies with a handful of nuts and raisins, air-popped popcorn, or fresh fruit. (For tips on what to eat for dinner, see pages 50–51.)

25. Lose that weight.

Obesity has been linked to insomnia, snoring, obstructive sleep apnea, and other sleep problems and disorders. If you are overweight, see your doctor and get started on a weight-loss program. Your sleep patterns—and your overall health—will reap dramatic benefits.

26. Tame your sweet tooth.

If you're into sugary foods, you probably have a hard time sleeping. That's because sugar tampers with your body chemistry and sends you into a Jekyll-and-Hyde tailspin. Say that you have a Danish in the morning on your way to work. The Danish gives you a brief hit of energy and euphoria . . . but then you come crashing down. You have another snack to get over the crash—maybe a doughnut or a cookie. More energy, more euphoria, then *whammo!* You crash again. The madness goes on all day long, until your body is completely out of whack and unable to get back to a natural cycle of restful sleep and energetic wakefulness. So the next time you're craving a sweet, reach for a healthier alternative like fresh or dried fruit, sugar-free instant pudding, or yogurt.

27. Hydrate.
Make sure to drink eight to ten glasses of water daily—more, if it's hot out or you engage in exercise. Staying properly hydrated is essential to good health. A tall glass of water may also give you the pick-me-up you need when you're feeling sluggish during the day.

28. Add foods rich in magnesium and thiamin (Vitamin B_1) to your diet.
Studies have shown that low levels of magnesium and thiamin may be related to insomnia. Foods high in magnesium include almonds, barley, quinoa, spinach, avocados, and oysters. Foods high in thiamin include fresh pasta, rice, wheat, tuna, salmon, pork, and asparagus.

29. Cut down on caffeine—or eliminate it altogether.
There's no question that caffeine consumption messes with our bodies—and with our sleep. Don't touch caffeine six hours or less before your bedtime, since that's how long it can stay in your system. (Some experts suggest that caffeine can stay in the

If you do decide to give up caffeine, do it gradually. Decrease your daily consumption a little at a time. Otherwise, you may experience withdrawal symptoms such as irritability and headaches.

system for as long as twelve hours.) And for the rest of the day, consider scaling down your caffeine consumption. Or, if you're really, really good and virtuous, consider giving it up altogether. My personal caffeine routine: one cup of tasty French roast at breakfast, and a cup of Earl Grey tea at three in the afternoon—like the English do.

Keep in mind that caffeine doesn't just come in a mug. It can also be found in cola-style soft drinks, chocolate, and some over-the-counter and prescription pills.

30. Stop smoking!

We all know that there are about eight hundred compelling reasons to quit smoking. We can add "good sleep" to the list. Studies have shown that smokers have a harder time going to sleep and waking up, and experience more sleep disturbances during the night. Also, heavy smokers often have respiratory problems, which can contribute to poor sleep. To stop smoking today, follow the excellent tips on the American Cancer Society's Web site: *www.cancer. org/tobacco/quitting.html.*

31. Get some sun.

If you spend a lot of time indoors—i.e., in an office—it's important to get a little sunlight every day. This will help adjust your internal clock so your mind and body will know the difference between night and day. Walk to and from work; grab a quick stroll at lunch; take mini-breaks to grab a strawberry smoothie, buy office supplies, run to the post office. If you're going to be outside for more than twenty minutes, make sure to slap on the sunblock (SPF15 or higher) fifteen to thirty minutes before you go out. (This rule applies even if it's overcast, early in the morning, or late in the day.)

32. Take a fifteen- to thirty-minute "power nap" in the afternoon.

Some sleep experts recommend a short nap about halfway between the time you wake up and go to sleep. This is the time when your internal circadian

> Each afternoon I go into the ladies' lounge at my office, curl up on the couch, and nap for fifteen minutes while listening to music on my headphones. At first the other women didn't get it. But now they're all vying for couch time so they can get their naps, too!
>
> —Stacy, age 32

rhythms naturally take a nosedive, which might explain that "can't-keep-your-eyes-open" feeling many people experience at this time of day. Instead of trying to tough it through the rest of the afternoon on espresso shots, try a nap instead. If you work in an office, close the door (if you have one), unplug the phone, and curl up on a comfy chair or put your head down on your desk. Make sure you don't nap for longer than thirty minutes, since this can send you into a deeper sleep state and make it harder for you to conk out at bedtime. (Note: Some people may find this to be the case with even a short afternoon nap. See what works for you.)

33. Exercise daily.
Studies have shown that a regular exercise regime can help you get to sleep—and stay asleep—by re-

leasing "feel-good" endorphin chemicals, fine-tuning your nighttime body temperature, keeping your weight down, and more. If you suffer from a medical condition, are overweight, or have not exercised in a long time, be sure to consult your doctor before starting an exercise program.

Here are some great ways to add exercise to your life:

- Walk instead of driving, whenever you can.

- Get a trial membership at your local gym and see if it's for you.

- Rediscover your bicycle and ride it everywhere.

- Sign up for cardio kickboxing classes.

- Take long, brisk walks with your dog.

- Dance! There's ballet, modern, tap, African, ballroom, Irish step, and so much more. (And of course, there's boogying in your living room.)

- Buy his-and-hers Rollerblades, helmets, and pads—then hit the trails *à deux*.

- Look into a Resista-Ball class—really terrific workouts for your entire body that involves rolling around on a huge ball.

- Swim.

- Fire the cleaning lady and the kid who mows your lawn and do these tasks yourself.

- Join a jogging club, a softball team, a tennis league.

- Buy a treadmill and use it while you watch TV.

34. Be a day owl.

Stay busy and active during the day so that you'll be naturally tired at bedtime. Clean your closets. Visit friends. Take up a new language. Read all those books you've been meaning to read. Volunteer. If you exercise your mind and give your goals a workout, you'll find yourself falling into a contented sleep when bedtime rolls around.

35. Take care of business.

Become efficient and organized so you can get the day's business done *during the day*. Knock off your errands, bills, and other chores during a set chunk

I used to be a major procrastinator. This would keep me up half the night because I'd stay up worrying about all the things I avoided doing. Now I shut off the Internet, close my door, let my secretary take my calls, and Do My Work. Since I'm now sleeping through the night, I'm heading to work refreshed and raring to go.

—Lois, age 42

of time (e.g., during a midmorning break or at lunch). Whatever you don't get done, put on your to-do list for tomorrow—*and don't think about it till tomorrow*. Ditto with work. Don't let the day's unfinished business spill over into your evening winddown time—or worse yet, your sleeping time.

36. Get stroked.

Massage promotes relaxation, relieves stress, enhances circulation and energy flow, and more. And the best part is, you get to lie there and enjoy it while someone else does the work! Ask your physician, friends, or local gym to refer you to a qualified massage therapist. Many day spas and hotels have massage therapists on staff. Rates will vary, but will probably range from forty to a hundred dollars an hour. Depending on where you live, you may be able to choose from a menu of options: Swedish massage (the most common type), shiatsu, Thai massage, sports massage, and more. (On the home front, you could buy some candles and scented oils and convince your honey to be your private massage therapist—for purely therapeutic reasons, of course.)

As the Sun Goes Down . . .

As night approaches and the world slows down, it's time for you to slow down, too. There are a number of things you should absolutely do during these hours . . . and a number of things you should absolutely *not* do.

37. Go easy on the liquor.

Drinking alcohol in the evening can lead to sleep problems. After a couple of beers at cocktail hour followed by margaritas with dinner, you may stumble into bed and go out like a light. But you will likely wake up a few hours later and not be able to go back to sleep. Or, your sleeping will be so shallow that you will feel exhausted the next day. Generally speaking, a glass of wine before or during dinner will probably not affect your sleep. But most experts agree that you should avoid having any alcohol within two or three hours of bedtime.

38. Don't eat dinner too close to bedtime.

You don't want your digestive system working overtime in the middle of the night and keeping you

> If I have a couple of martinis at happy hour, I find myself waking up at four in the morning and staring at the ceiling till my alarm goes off. Ugh!
>
> —Sonja, age 29

awake. Eat dinner on the early side so your metabolism can wind down. If you are at a party and neither the serving hour nor the menu is in your control, remember that portion size and food selection are choices you make—so choose wisely.

39. Try tryptophan.

A turkey sandwich for dinner may be just what you need for sweet dreams later. Turkey—and also chicken, fish, meat, eggs, dairy products, soybeans, nuts, and seeds—all contain a substance known as tryptophan, which has proven sleep-inducing properties. Adding carbs (such as pasta or bread) will help your body absorb the tryptophan.

40. Exercise is great—but don't do it too late.

A daily workout program is essential to good sleep, but try not to exercise too close to bedtime. Some experts say you shouldn't engage in vigorous exer-

---

Keep up your healthy eating regime at dinnertime.
Stick to lean meats or fish, grains, veggies, and pasta
(modest helpings, please, and no heavy, creamy, or
oily sauces). Roasting, steaming, and poaching are
definitely preferable to frying of any kind.

---

cise up to six hours before bedtime—some say
three. See what works for you.

41. Take an after-dinner stroll.
A nice family walk (or a nice alone-time walk)
should not fall into the prohibited "vigorous exercise" category for most people—so go for it! Furthermore, it can aid your digestion, promote
relaxation, and get you in the mood for sleep.

42. Have a winding-down ritual.
Start unwinding early in the evening, preferably
right after your walk. This will send a message to
your mind and body that they should be transition-
ing from active day mode to sleepy night mode.
Your winding-down ritual could include: listening
to classical music or jazz; writing in your journal;
giving yourself an at-home beauty treatment (think
facials, manicures, pedicures); setting out your

> I can't get to the gym until 9:30 P.M. It is also the
> time when most of the machines are free. The late
> hour may be a problem for some people, but once
> I get home, I sleep like a baby.
>
> —Christine, age 36

clothes for tomorrow; talking on the phone with
your best buds; reading a novel.

43. Censor your TV-watching.

If your winding-down ritual includes TV, steer clear
of violent or disturbing shows, including the news.
They will wind you up rather than wind you down
and make it harder to fall asleep later.

44. Clear the air with your partner.

If you and your partner have an argument coming,
have it out now. Bedtime is not the time—and your
marital bed is not the place—to fight. So sit down
and air your grievances now, or make an appointment—that's right, an *appointment*—for a time tomorrow that would be more convenient to hash stuff
out.

> At 9 P.M., no matter how swamped I am, I drop everything and curl up in my favorite chair with a cup of chamomile tea and a magazine. It's my little escape, and it helps me relax so I can get to sleep later.
>
> —Elizabeth, age 34

45. Make a "tomorrow list."

If you have any leftover worries or anxieties from the day, write them down on a piece of paper and promise yourself that you'll take care of them tomorrow. That's *tomorrow*—not tonight, while you're tossing and turning in bed. Then tuck that piece of paper into your day calendar and stop thinking about it. Remind yourself that you will be able to tackle your problems more effectively after a good night's sleep.

46. Practice yoga and meditation.

Both yoga and meditation are wonderful ways to de-stress, decompress, and improve your overall health—all of which will help you get quality sleep. Sign up for classes or pick up a book or videotape.

> I've been sleeping a whole lot better since I've
> adopted my new mantra: *I can't do anything about
> it now. It can wait till tomorrow.*
>
> —Angela, age 41

(Both yoga and meditation are also terrific things to
do earlier in the day—or right before you go to bed.)

47. Start anticipating your bedtime with pleasure.

As the sun goes down and you're winding down,
enjoy the thought that in just a few short hours, you
can slip into your cozy, wonderful bed.

Time for Bed!

Bedtime can all too often consist of putting a pile of work aside ("Oops, didn't realize it was so late!"), brushing one's teeth, throwing on a pair of pajamas, and flopping into bed. No wonder so many people can't fall asleep!

Here are some tips to help you ease gently into the arms of Morpheus.

48. Try to go to bed at the same time every night, even on weekends.

This isn't as crucial as waking up at the same time every morning. However, having a regular bedtime will make it easier to fall asleep at night. Yes, you have to go dancing till 3 A.M. once in a while . . . and yes, I know it's hard to turn off the late-night movie when Harry is just about to kiss Sally. But in general, and if possible, stick to a schedule.

49. Go to bed when you're drowsy.

Are you in the habit of going to bed at a certain time—say, when your partner likes to turn in, or

after your favorite ten-o'clock TV show—then find
yourself unable to fall asleep? Part of the problem
may be that you're *just not sleepy*. It's important to
go to bed when your internal schedule says "bedtime!" To move things along, follow the tips in the
rest of the chapter to help you get all noodly and
sleepy. (Note: If you get into a routine of waking
up at the same time every day, you will probably
find yourself getting drowsy at about the same time
every evening—which is a good thing.)

50. Give yourself permission to go to bed.

Many of us think of sleep as an afterthought, a thing
to be squeezed in, a low-priority item on the to-do
list of life. So when nine, ten, or eleven o'clock rolls
around, we feel as if we have to knock off a few
more essential chores before we're "allowed" to quit
and turn in for the night. Tonight, when you're bedtime rolls around, grant yourself permission to go to
bed. Then do it.

51. Do some gentle stretches.

It's important to get the day's kinks and aches out
of your muscles so you're not bothered by them in
the middle of the night. Before turning in, lie down
on a soft rug, on your bed, or on an exercise mat
and stretch your arms, your legs, your whole body.

Stretching hamstrings is important. Pain and tension from these muscles can keep people awake without them realizing that this is the source of discomfort. I also take magnesium tablets, which eliminate nagging muscle pain. Calcium/magnesium tablets do the same, plus they add a natural calming effect.

—Jeremy, age 52

Turn onto your side, then extend your arms and point your toes in opposite directions. Grow long, longer, longest. Do the same thing standing flat on your feet.

52. Do a last-minute check around the house.

Go around and make sure doors are locked, windows are secured, appliances are off, the smoke alarm is going, and children and pets are where they're supposed to be. Feeling safe and secure is crucial to getting a good night's sleep. While you're at it, tend to other little last-minute details: adjust the thermostat; make sure the humidifier, dehumidifier, or air conditioner is running as needed; pop a tape into the VCR to record favorite late-night shows; lay out your clothes for tomorrow; program your coffeemaker for the morning; take care of your pets' food, water, and "bathroom" needs.

53. Unplug the phone.

There's nothing like being woken up at midnight by a wrong number, a drunk ex, or a relative in another time zone. If you must have the telephone on for emergency purposes, turn the volume way down so you can't be bothered by an incoming call.

54. Take a warm bath.

A long, luxurious soak is a time-honored way to make yourself seriously (and blissfully) sleepy. Just before going to bed, slip into the tub and add lavender bath salts for an extra-sedative effect. Or get some Float Away sleep-enhancing milk bath from Origins (*www.origins.com*). A hot tub or Jacuzzi works wonders, too. (Of course, if you are pregnant or have a medical condition that might make super-hot bathing out of the question, check with your doctor first.)

55. Dress (or undress) appropriately for sleep.

Of course you should wear whatever you want to bed, whether it's a cute little nightie, flannel jams, a big comfy T-shirt, or nothing at all. Just make sure your nightclothes aren't too scratchy, constricting,

> My boyfriend and I take a bath together every night before we go to bed. He turns off all the lights in the apartment, and we light candles in the bathroom (for the bath) and the bedroom (for when we get into our pj's afterward). It's our way of telling ourselves and each other that it's bedtime. No more work, no more TV—it's just our bath and the candles and each other.
>
> —Elise, age 40

heavy, light, or otherwise uncomfortable. As for sleeping in the buff: Yes, it's sexy and it's intimate, but make sure you're not waking up chilled in the middle of the night and groping in the dark for blankets. Also, if you're prone to cold feet, don't forget the fuzzy socks.

56. Have a cozy nightcap.
Pass on the snifter of brandy or late-night Bud and go for a mug of warm milk (which is rich in tryptophan, as we learned on page 50). Other sleepy beverages include chamomile or valerian tea. A caveat: Skip this tip if drinking beverages in the evening makes you have to get up to go to the bathroom in the middle of the night.

Never use alcohol as a sleeping aid.

57. Make it a rule: The bed is only for sleeping and sex.

Your bed is a sacred space. Make it clear to yourself and to any sleeping companions that there will be no eating, drinking, bill paying, working, or surfing.

58. Then have sex.

Remember that thing about not having vigorous exercise up to six hours before bedtime? The one exception is sex. Pleasurable sexual activity, either alone or with a partner, can help you relax, fall asleep, and stay asleep. And of course, feel free to have sex the rest of the day, too—the more pleasure and relaxation in your life, the better! Think of it as "doctor's orders."

59. Put a few drops of lavender essential oil on your pillow.

Lavender has natural sedative properties that will help you get a deep, restful sleep. Look for little bottles of lavender essential oil at a natural-food store, a spa, or a reliable on-line source. My favorite:

On a stressful night when I feel tense, I might take a hot shower and drink a cup of hot milk with honey and go under my warm blanket.

—Ellen, age 37

Sweet Dreams Blend from Earth Tribe International (*www.earth-tribe.com*), which contains both lavender and marjoram. You can also purchase diffusers, aromatherapy balls, or other devices to release relaxing scents into the air.

60. Rub yourself with sleepy potions.

You can also put lavender oils, lotions, and other products right on your body to help you get to sleep. Browse the cosmetics section of your local health-food store. Or check out the Origins Web site at *www.origins.com* for their line of relaxing products, which includes Call It a Night sleep-deepening body lotion and Sleep Time on-the-spot gel.

61. Have your honey read you a bedtime story.

Why should there be an age limit on bedtime stories? Tonight, grab a copy of Mother Goose, *Chronicles of Narnia,* a book of Irish fairy tales, or other favorite volume and ask your significant other to

I need to sleep with a soft pillow over my ear (an old habit from living in the noisy city).
—Fiona, age 44

read you to sleep. Tomorrow, return the favor. If you're sleeping solo, consider a book on tape.

62. Banish the pets.
Yes, it's fun to cuddle with Muffy or Fido while you sleep. For some people pets can even be like security blankets. But they can also disturb your rest. Unless they're going to keep you up *more* by meowing or barking at the bedroom door, put them in another room for the night—preferably a faraway room.

63. Tune it out.
If you're especially sensitive to noise, and the noise-mitigating tips on pages 27–28 aren't enough for you, then this is the time to don a pair of good old-fashioned earplugs. Earplugs can be purchased in most drugstores.

64. Relax your body.
As you're trying to fall asleep, make a conscious effort to turn your body into Jell-O. Some proven techniques:

▪ Inhale on a count of eight. Hold your breath in for a count of eight. Exhale on a count of eight. Hold your breath out for a count of eight. Repeat.

▪ Tense the muscles in your toes for ten seconds, then untense them and breathe deeply for ten seconds. Move up your body and repeat this with all the muscle groups.

▪ Simultaneously tense all the muscles in your body—or as many as you can, anyway. Clench and squeeze like mad. Then release everything all at once and take a deep breath. Repeat.

▪ Picture your right arm. Picture it feeling very limp and noodly and relaxed. Imagine directing your breath into your right arm while you're doing this. Then move onto another part of your body. Continue doing this until your entire body is very limp and noodly and relaxed.

65. Relax your mind.
As you're trying to fall asleep, it's equally important to turn your mind into Jell-O. Here's how:

▪ Count sheep . . . or horses . . . or dancing fruit . . . or whatever works for you.

Falling asleep has never really been a problem for me, but when my mind is particularly preoccupied or I'm not able to drop off as soon as my head hits the pillow, I start counting, very slowly, backward from ten. With each number, I breathe deeply and try to relax more of the muscles in my body. Many times, I'll think I'm already relaxed, but then with each breath, I find more muscles that are still tense. I rarely have reached zero without falling asleep.

—Sarah, age 32

▪ Re-create your favorite memories—your first date with your spouse, graduation day, Game Six of the '86 World Series—and play them over in your head, detail by detail.

▪ Listen to a tape of soothing music or natural noises: waves, falling rain, tropical birds.

▪ Write a short story or screenplay in your head. Start with a character, put her in the middle of a not-too-intense conflict (girl loses boy; girl loses favorite pair of shoes; girl loses way in downtown Newark), then get her out of it.

▪ Imagine yourself on a lush Caribbean beach. You're lying on the sand . . . the waves tickle your

> I play out chess games in my head. The effort of remembering and visualizing the positions puts me to sleep.
>
> —Mark, age 44

toes . . . the salty breeze caresses your skin. All you hear are the shushing of the waves and the voice of the cabana boy softly murmuring, "Would you like another piña colada?" Mmmmmm.

66. Chase away upsetting thoughts.

As you're drifting off with visions of sheep or piña coladas dancing in your head, unwelcome visions may intrude: that stack of unpaid bills, your boss yelling about deadlines, the dry cleaning you forgot to pick up. If this happens, try this trick: Put the image or thought in a fluffy white cloud and watch the cloud drift away—slowly, slowly—across a bright blue sky. If the image or thought returns, repeat the exercise. At no point should you beat up on yourself because you "keep thinking about negative stuff." Just focus on that cloud.

67. Get in position.

Sleeping on your side may be the best bet—but make sure your pillow is placed in such a way as to

Sometimes, when I can't sleep, I pretend that I have to pull an all-nighter to get a paper done—but that I'm just going to lie down and close my eyes for a second before I get started. I fall right to sleep.

—Jasmine, age 22

align your head with the rest of your body. If you tend to snore, you may not want to sleep on your back. Sleeping on your stomach can lead to head-aches, neck aches, and backaches.

68. Don't put your head under your pillow or covers.

Yes, this can be a tempting way to tune out the outside world. But covering your head can diminish your oxygen supply and give you a massive middle-of-the-night headache.

69. If you can't fall asleep after fifteen minutes, get up and do something else.

But don't do something that's fun that's going to keep you up such as watching TV or reading your favorite magazine. Do something monotonous—maybe water plants or read junk mail. Return to bed only when you're tired.

70. Don't stew.

If you can't fall asleep, don't lie there stressing out about the fact that you can't fall sleep. The mental agitation will only compound your insomnia. Instead, go back to the tips number 65 and 66, and work on relaxing your body and mind.

71. Try to stay awake.

Call it "reverse psychology" or "paradoxical intent." Some people find that if they try to stay awake while lying in bed, they'll drift off *just like that*.

72. Keep it dark.

Candles and pretty lamps (with or without colored bulbs) can provide just the right atmosphere for evening winding-down time. But from the time you fall asleep to the time you wake up, it's important to keep it as dark as possible. That means all candles and lamps must be off, and no lights should leak in from adjoining rooms. If safety is a concern—i.e., you need to be able to find the bathroom at 2 A.M., or your children need to be able to find *you* at 2 A.M.—consider one or two small night-lights that plug into outlets. If you're particularly light-sensitive, you might consider extra-heavy, opaque drapes for your windows. A night mask—available in drugstores—is also a good option.

If You're Up in the Middle of the Night

It's awful to wake up in the middle of the night and not be able to go back to sleep. You stare at the ceiling. You stare at the blinking numbers on the alarm clock (3:01, 3:02, 3:03, 3:04, 3:05 . . . and then, a little later, it's 4:00, 4:01, 4:02, 4:03). You stare at your slumbering partner—how can they sleep so peacefully while you lie there tossing and turning?

A crucial component of good sleep is *continuous* sleep. This will ensure that you go through all the appropriate sleep stages, including frequent—and extended—REM (Rapid Eye Movement) stages. This, in turn, will ensure that you wake up feeling rested, restored, and ready to go.

Here are some tips to beat the midnight-to-dawn insomnia vigil. And remember: Many of the tips in the previous section will help you at 3 A.M. as well as at 10 P.M.

73. Figure out what woke you up.
Are you hungry? Thirsty? Do you have to go to the bathroom? Are you too cold, too hot, too cramped?

When I toss around in bed and cannot fall asleep because of bad thoughts, I try to make up a story in my head, usually an adventure story with me as a protagonist in a faraway land. I usually fall asleep before the happy end.

—Faith, age 37

Pinpoint the source of your wakefulness and deal with it immediately—while you're still sleepy.

74. Clear your head.

If you woke up because you're anxious about the report that's due tomorrow or because you feel bad about the fight you had with your friend, make a conscious effort to chase those thoughts away. Tell yourself that everything will turn out fine—tomorrow. Then occupy your mind with sheep or clouds or other mindless, distracting, drowsy-making images.

75. Write it down.

You wake up in a sweat: Oh no, did you forget to mail the rent check? Was it your mother's birthday yesterday? For such occasions, keep a notebook and pen on your nightstand so you can write down any red flags that pop up in the wee hours. That way you won't lie there tossing and turning and wondering if you'll remember to do this stuff tomorrow.

76. Train your bladder.

Having to get up in the middle of the night to go to the bathroom is a common obstacle to continuous, restful sleep. Remember to limit alcoholic intake in the evenings. Some people prefer not to drink anything at all—even water—after 4, 5, or 6 P.M. See what works for you. Also, unless it's extremely uncomfortable or medically unwise (e.g., because of a prostate or bladder condition), you might consider ignoring "nature's call" and trying to get back to sleep.

77. If you have to go to the bathroom, aim in the dark.

If you *do* have to go to the bathroom in the middle of the night, avoid turning on any lights, which will confuse your internal clock. ("Is it day or is it night or what?") Have a few discreetly placed night-lights in the hallway and bathroom instead. In general, avoid turning on lights in the middle of the night unless it is absolutely necessary.

78. Talk yourself down from a nightmare.

Monsters . . . bad guys with guns chasing you . . . airplane crashes. You sit up in bed, you're drenched in sweat, your heart is racing a mile a minute, and you're wide wake. Instead of letting the nightmare control you, control *it*. Get into a comfortable position and take some deep, cleansing breaths. Tell yourself that it's *just a dream*. Mentally rewrite the same dream so that you win in the end. Replace the bad dream with pleasant fantasies.

79. Put the lid on snoring.

Snoring—your own or your partner's—can wake you up in the middle of the night. If the snoring seems excessive or causes you or your partner to stop breathing periodically, check with your family doctor to rule out obstructive sleep apnea, hypertension, or other problems. If it's just garden-variety snoring, here are some trips to keep it at bay:

▪ Lose weight and get in shape. Flabby muscles in the throat and jaw area can lead to snoring.

▪ Don't sleep on your back. Some people sew golf balls into the back pockets of their pajamas in order to "train" themselves not to roll onto their backs.

> Whenever I'm up in the middle of the night and can't get back to sleep, I play this mind game with myself. I pretend that it's 6 A.M. and the alarm has gone off and my kids are bugging me to wake up and make them breakfast. I think, "No, I don't want to get up yet, just let me sleep for five more minutes!" I conk right out.
>
> —Ruth, age 45

- Reduce nasal congestion. A stuffy nose can intensify snoring.

- Make sure your bedroom isn't too dry. Use a humidifier, if necessary.

- Avoid sleeping pills, antihistamines, alcohol, and snacks several hours before bedtime.

- Don't smoke!

- Talk to your doctor. He or she can advise you about surgical procedures and devices to alleviate snoring.

80. Be wary of so-called antisnoring products.
This includes pillows, nasal sprays, herbal pills, jaw retainers, and more. None of them have been proven

scientifically to work, despite what the ads may say. The exception is a nasal dilator called Breathe Right, which has been approved by the FDA. If you're not sure about Breathe Right or any other product, ask your doctor.

81. Don't obsess about being awake.

It's important not to lie there thinking: "I'm awake . . . This is really going to screw up my day tomorrow . . . Is it really 2:45 A.M.? . . . What is wrong with me, anyway?" Relax, take some deep breaths, and take the work out of sleeping. Just enjoy lying there in your soft, comfy bed, in the dark, with no cares or obligations in the world. Don't stare at the ceiling or the clock. Tell yourself how nice it is that you have many, many more hours of pure, luxurious rest till you have to get up and start your busy day.

Family Matters

It's one thing to get a good night's sleep if you're living alone—or with a quiet, unobtrusive sleeping partner. It's another thing altogether if you have a newborn in the house . . . or young children . . . or a partner who seems to live in a different time zone from you, or who otherwise disrupts your snoozing schedule.

Here are some tips to help you get your zzz's when your family keeps you from getting the sleep you dearly need.

82. If you have a newborn, keep nighttime activity to a minimum.

Of course you have to feed the baby or change the baby's diaper in the middle of the night. But keep the lights out or on low while you do this; perform these tasks quickly and efficiently; and don't excite the baby with singing, music, toys, or happy chatter. The sooner your baby realizes the difference between nighttime (sleeptime!) and daytime (playtime!), the better.

83. If possible, have someone else tend to the baby in the middle of the night.

You'll have a better chance of continuous rest if family members take turns feeding, changing, and otherwise taking care of the baby during the midnight-to-dawn shift. If you're nursing, use a breast pump and freeze your breast milk in sterile plastic bags or bottles. They can be thawed quickly in the microwave or a bowl of hot water.

84. Make your children follow the same sleep strategies as you.

Many of the tips in the previous chapters apply to your children as well. Among other things, it's crucial that your children have healthy diets; fresh air and exercise; a regular wake-up time; winding-down time at night; and a regular bedtime.

85. Create safe, snug, comfortable bedroom environments for your children.

As with your bedroom, your children's bedrooms should be cool but not cold (around sixty-five degrees) and not too dry or humid. A night-light can make them feel secure, as can leaving the door open. Make sure they have good beds and bedding. Encourage them to cuddle with a stuffed animal in the

> Every night at around eight o'clock, the kids and I
> get into our pajamas, climb onto the couch, turn the
> lights down low, and read a bedtime story. It makes
> them sleepy. And it makes me sleepy, too!
>
> —Marybeth, age 41

middle of the night (instead of tiptoeing into your bedroom and waking you up).

86. Keep nightmares at bay.

Young children are very susceptible to nightmares. They also have a hard time distinguishing reality from fantasy. Don't allow them to watch scary TV before going to bed (or, for that matter, don't let them watch scary TV at all). This includes adult TV shows and local or national news. Read only soothing and happy bedtime stories to them—nothing with slimy monsters or flesh-eating dinosaurs.

87. Consider the pros and cons of a "family bed."

Some families believe in the family bed, where Mom, Dad, babies, young kids, and older kids are welcome to sleep. A bunch of beds can be pushed together in one room to accommodate especially large families. Proponents argue that this practice not only promotes closeness, but prevents middle-of-the-night wakings because everyone is right there: Mom doesn't have to get up to nurse the baby; little children can find instant comfort and cuddling if they have a nightmare.

Opponents argue that the whole family sleeping together can actually lead to more sleep disruptions and long-term sleep problems.

Some good pro-family-bed books include: *The Family Bed* by Tina Thevenin and *Three in a Bed: The Benefits of Sharing Your Bed with Your Baby* by Deborah Jackson and Tom Newton.

88. Consider separate beds.

Does your partner snore, grind his or her teeth, thrash around, mumble, or otherwise keep you up at night? First try earplugs or a bigger bed. Make him or her read this book and follow all the tips. But if all else fails, you might consider separate beds—or if necessary, separate bedrooms.

89. Accept your and your mate's biological clock.

Maybe your mate likes to stay up till the wee hours and get up at noon—whereas you can't keep your eyes open past 9 P.M., and you're rarin' to go at

> When I was pregnant, I had lots of backaches because of my big stomach. My husband massaged my back every night before we went to bed. He would put on a soothing CD, light a candle, and use vanilla-scented oil. It made it so much easier to fall asleep!
>
> —Anna, age 28

dawn. These preferences may actually be genetically determined, which means there's not a whole lot you can do to change them. Try to work around each other's schedule—and make sure your mate's awake-time activities don't keep you up (and vice versa). Take comfort in the fact that things may change as you get older—elderly people tend to be morning people.

90. If you're pregnant, hug a pillow.

Speaking of family matters: Pregnancy can present special challenges for sleep. Hormones are raging . . . you have to go to the bathroom about twelve times a night . . . your stomach is so gosh-darned *huge*. And it's hard not to stew and worry about how your world is going to be turned upside down in a few short months when the baby comes—agggh!

It's very important for pregnant women to follow the tips in this book. There are also extra-long, body-length pillows made especially to help pregnant women sleep. Wrap your arms and legs around it . . . let it support your belly. You can buy these pillows on-line at *www.stillworks.com, www.amazon.com*, or *www.sleepmatterzzz.com*. Pregnancy massage can also help.

Last but Not Least

Hopefully the previous ninety tips have helped you get the zzz's you need. Here are some final ones to cover some special topics—jet lag and shift work, for example—and also address important sleep-related issues like herbal remedies, sleeping pills, sleep disorders, and more.

91. Don't let jet lag drag you down.
Jet lag can throw off your internal clock and make getting a good night's sleep a nightmare. To avoid jet lag—or to lessen its effects—follow these guide-lines:

▪ If possible, avoid red-eye flights and early, early morning flights. Also avoid flights that will get you to your destination past your bedtime.

▪ Start adjusting your internal clock before your trip so you can get a leg up. If you're flying west, start staying up and getting up later a few days before your trip. If you're flying east, do the opposite.

▪ Reduce travel stress by planning and preparing for your trip in a timely fashion. Don't rush to the airport at the last minute.

▪ When you get on the plane, immediately set your watch for the time it is in your destination. If you're flying from New York City to L.A., and it's noon when you take off, you should set your watch for 9 A.M.—and start pretending immediately that it's 9 A.M. where you are. During the course of your flight and after you reach your destination, follow your new schedule—e.g., eat lunch at L.A. time and not at New York time.

▪ On the plane, drink plenty of water to keep yourself hydrated. Avoid alcohol. Also avoid cigarettes and heavy or spicy foods.

▪ Take frequent walks up and down the aisles. Do gentle stretching at your seat.

▪ Once you reach your destination, use daylight to help you adjust to your new time zone. Expose yourself to the sun by taking lots of walks.

92. Stay on schedule.

While you're traveling—whether for business or pleasure—try to stay on the wake-up and bedtime schedule you normally follow (according to whatever time zone you're in, that is). Continue to follow the tips in this book, including limiting alcohol intake, getting regular exercise, and eating an early, *healthy* dinner.

93. If you do shift work, pay special attention to your sleep needs.

Shift work can present special challenges for people—especially if their shift changes frequently. If you're a shift worker:

▪ As with plane travel, try to adjust to your shift schedule as far in advance as possible. For example, if you have a night shift coming up, try to go to bed a little later each evening and wake up later each morning.

▪ Establish a regular eating schedule for the duration of your shift. Eat meals and snacks at about the same time.

▪ Likewise, establish a regular sleep schedule for the duration of your shift.

▪ Avoid coffee and other caffeinated products at the end of your shift, or you won't be able to fall asleep for many hours after you get home.

• If you're getting off a night shift, avoid drinking alcohol after work. It will make it harder for you to sleep during the day. Wear dark glasses during the drive home so that your internal clock isn't confused by the daylight. Make sure your bedroom at home is cool and dark, and remove all possible sources of noise. Unplug the phone; put up "Do Not Disturb" signs; talk to your family beforehand about leaving you in peace.

• If you experience serious or prolonged sleep, health, or other problems as a result of your shift work, be sure to consult a doctor.

94. Pay off your sleep debt as soon as possible.
Yes, once in a while, you're going to pull an all-nighter to meet a deadline . . . or stay up partying till dawn . . . or get your after-dinner caf and decaf mixed up and find yourself staring at your alarm clock till the wee hours. Just be sure to make up for your bad night's sleep as soon as possible—by returning to your normal, eight-hours-a-night-plus sleep schedule and staying there. Do not try to compensate for your bad night with lots of caffeine and sugary snacks the next day. These quick-hit solutions will only send you crashing, mess up your in-

> After a night of zero sleep, I used to use coffee to get me through the next day. But it only made it worse. I was a wreck all day and I wouldn't be able to sleep the next night. Now, if I get bad sleep, I drink lots of water and freshly squeezed orange juice the next day. I actually have more energy that way, and I can sleep at night.
>
> —Karen, age 34

ternal clock further, and prolong the effects of your sleep deprivation.

95. Start keeping a sleep diary.
In order to sleep better, it's important to be aware of your sleep patterns. Starting tomorrow, make a note of the following every day:

- the time you woke up

- how you felt when you woke up (e.g., exhausted, groggy, energetic)

- how many hours you slept

- how many times you woke up during the night

- whether you exercised

- whether you ate healthy meals

- whether you had alcohol or caffeine during the evening

- what time you went to bed

- any stressful events during the day

Feel free to custom-tailor your sleep diary any way you see fit. Over several weeks, you should be able to make a general assessment of your sleep patterns, your potential trouble areas, and so forth.

96. If this book hasn't helped you start sleeping better—or if you suspect that you have a sleep disorder—then consult your doctor or a sleep clinic.

As you know by now, sleep deprivation is no laughing matter. If nothing is working for you, or if you think you might be suffering from a sleep disorder, call your doctor. He or she may be able to treat you, or may refer you to a sleep clinic that specializes in sleep issues.

Here is a rundown of the most common sleep disorders:

■ *Insomnia:* This is what most of this book has been about. Insomnia can be a stand-alone condition or a symptom of another sleep disorder, an underlying physical or psychological illness, or a medication side effect. It includes these problems: trouble falling asleep at night; waking up in the middle of the night and tossing and turning; waking up too early in the morning and not being able to get back to sleep; and waking up feeling tired and unrefreshed. Self-care measures (such as the ones described in this book) may or may not work for insomnia, depending on its cause.

■ *Obstructive Sleep Apnea:* This is a disorder characterized by loud snoring and actual cessations in breathing due to the throat muscles failing to stay open during sleep. It can have serious consequences for the person's health, and can be potentially life-threatening. Overweight people are at higher risk for sleep apnea. More men develop it than women. Mild cases can be treated with medications or pumplike devices that facilitate breathing—or simply by losing weight or sleeping on one's side. More serious cases may require surgery.

▪ *Restless Leg Syndrome:* Those with RLS find it seemingly impossible to keep their legs still while lying down. There can be aching, itching, tingling, or other uncomfortable sensations that make the desire to move the legs almost irresistible. Many RLS sufferers can find relief only by getting up in the middle of the night and walking around. RLS can be hereditary. Treatment usually involves prescription medication along with relaxation therapy.

▪ *Periodic Limb Movement Disorder:* This disorder is similar to RLS, except that most of the leg movements occur during sleep. Many people who have RLS can also have periodic limb movement disorder. The treatment courses are similar.

▪ *Parasomnia:* Parasomnia is an umbrella term for a group of disorders that are characterized by strange, unsleeplike behavior during sleep. An estimated 2-million-plus people suffer from parasomnia. Examples include cooking and eating an entire meal while asleep, going on a cleaning binge, or having sex. The sleeper wakes up later with no awareness of having engaged in these activities. Sleepwalking and bruxism (see below) fall into this category.

- *Sleepwalking:* Sleepwalking, or somnambulism, can involve anything from sitting up in bed to walking to traveling long distances—all without waking up. One should not wake a sleepwalker unless it's an absolute emergency.

- *Bruxism:* Bruxism is a sleep disorder characterized by chronic teeth grinding during sleep. It is often caused by stress. Consult your dentist if you think you suffer from bruxism; he or she can recommend a plastic tooth guard for you to wear at night. Relaxation therapy can also help.

97. Check out alternative therapies.
Acupuncture, hypnosis, and other alternative therapies are sometimes used to treat insomnia. Consult your doctor or a sleep clinic for information and referrals.

98. Be careful about sleeping pills.
Yes, sleeping pills—whether the over-the-counter or prescription variety—may have their uses in certain situations. But they can also be addictive and pose side effects. Try the self-help measures in this book first. If you feel that sleeping pills are necessary, talk

to your doctor about the pros and cons and make an informed decision. In any case, they should be a short-term—not long-term—solution.

99. Likewise, approach herbal and other natural remedies with caution.

"Herbal" and "natural" are not synonymous with "safe" or "side effect–free." Herbal and other natural remedies are powerful medicines, and must be approached with the appropriate respect—and caution. Furthermore, they are not regulated by the FDA. There are a number of herbs and other natural substances that are used as sleep aids: valerian, melatonin, 5-HTP, and GABA (gamma-aminobutyric acid), just to name a few. Some are used alone; some are used in conjunction with each other or other substances. For helpful information on herbal and other natural remedies (e.g., their effectiveness, recommended doses, potential side effects, and more) check out a bookstore for informational guides or look up the Whole Health MD Web site at *www.wholehealthmd.com/hc/insomnia/ supplements/*. Also talk to your doctor about them.

100. Change your attitude about sleep.

So many of us think of sleep in negative terms: as a tedious necessity . . . as a biological force that

> For me, I think of sleep the way I think of facials.
> It's so lovely and luxurious, and I wake up looking
> great. What could be better?
>
> —Rosalie, age 29

drags down our minds and bodies . . . as a passive event that takes us away from other, more productive activities. Start thinking about sleep as a *positive* thing. Remember that good sleep is a necessity—as much as food, water, and air—to keep you at your peak physically, emotionally, mentally, professionally, and more. On top of which, sleep is pure, lazy pleasure. You should look forward to it at the end of each day as much as you'd look forward to a day at the beach.

101. Put sleep at the top of you list.

Decide—starting today!—that good sleep is going to be a priority in your life. Good sleep should be as important a goal as losing weight, starting an exercise program, getting a raise, or spending more time with a significant other. In fact, if you begin sleeping better, your other goals are sure to become more attainable because of your increased energy, improved mood, and more.

If it's daytime, read this book again, cover to cover—and start experiencing better sleep tonight.

If it's bedtime, put this book aside and get to bed. Sweet dreams!

APPENDIX

Helpful Resources

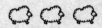

- **The National Sleep Foundation**
  (*www.sleepfoundation.org*)

- **The American Academy of Sleep Medicine**
  (*www.aasmnet.org*)

- **The National Center for Sleep Disorders**
  (*www.nhlbi.nih.gov/about/ncsdr*)

- **The Better Sleep Council**
  (*www.bettersleep.org*)

Nancy Butcher writes and edits health-related subjects on the World Wide Web. She is also the author of *101 Ways to Stop Eating After Dinner* and *How to Make Your Man Look Good (Without Making Him Feel Bad)*.

PENGUIN PUTNAM INC.
Online
Your Internet gateway to a virtual environment with
hundreds of entertaining and enlightening books
from Penguin Putnam Inc.

*While you're there, get the latest buzz on
the best authors and books around—*

Tom Clancy, Patricia Cornwell, W.E.B. Griffin,
Nora Roberts, William Gibson, Robin Cook,
Brian Jacques, Catherine Coulter, Stephen King,
Ken Follett, Terry McMillan, and many more!

**Penguin Putnam Online is located at
http://www.penguinputnam.com**

PENGUIN PUTNAM NEWS
Every month you'll get an inside look at our upcom-
ing books and new features on our site. This is an
ongoing effort to provide you with the most
up-to-date information about
our books and authors.

**Subscribe to Penguin Putnam News at
http://www.penguinputnam.com/newsletters**